1

TABLE OF CONTENTS

THIS BOOK IS TRANSLATED FROM GERMAN: VITAMIN D: WIRKUNGEN AUF DEN MENSCHLICHEN KÖRPER- AUF BASIS AKTUELLER WISSENSCHAFTLICHER ERKENNTNISSE KINDLE AUSGABE, CHRISOTPHER SCHÜTZE, VIENNA, ASUTRIA, 2019

Summary:

Despite numerous reports of the association of vitamin D with a spectrum of development, disease treatment and maintenance of health, vitamin D deficiency is common. (1) Severe vitamin D deficiency can cause rickets in infants or children and osteomalacia in adults. (2) However, this is currently rare in industrialized countries. (1, 2) Nevertheless, subclinical vitamin D deficiency is more common and has been reported to be associated with osteoporosis and a higher incidence of falls or fractures. (1) It has been reported that 96% of children with rickets were breastfed, as breast milk contains insufficient vitamin D. (1, 2) Since vitamin D receptors are present throughout the body, inadequate vitamin D status may be associated with several extra-skeletal effects, such as pregnancy-related complications and immunodeficiency. (1) It is well known that vitamin D can be obtained by exposure to sunlight or natural food sources. (2) The American Academy of Dermatology has classified ultraviolet radiation as a known skin carcinogen. (2) Therefore, it may not be safe or effective to receive vitamin D by sun exposure. (2) Hence, many paediatricians and physicians recommend adequate vitamin D supplementation to achieve optimal plasma concentrations. (1, 2) Most of the population suffers from vitamin D deficiency, especially in the winter months. (1) Studies have reported that vitamin D deficiency may play a role in the pathogenesis and / or progression of multiple diseases. (1) The widespread lack of vitamin D therefore deserves consideration, including raising public awareness and health professionals. (1-7) This book summarizes important mechanisms of action of vitamin D in the human body based on current scientific findings.

Introduction:

Rickets, a disease with impaired mineralization of bone tissue, can result in weak bones in infants and children. The disease is characterized by impaired bone mineralization. (7) The word "rickets" was first used in 1634. (3) Reports from the Royal Infirmary in Manchester indicate that cod liver oil has a beneficial effect on rickets. (1) In 1822 Sniadecki pointed to the relationship between sunlight and rickets. (4) At the end of the First World War, when rickets was an untreatable major problem in Vienna, Harriet Chick led a group of the British Medical Research Council to conduct research into this. (5) It was suggested that both cod liver oil and sunlight could cure rickets. In 1922, McCollum et al. termed "vitamin D" in publications, indicating the existence of a vitamin that promotes calcium deposition. (6)

1,25-dihydroxyvitamin D (1,25 (OH) 2D3) is the active form of vitamin D and activates the vitamin D receptor (VDR). VDR is a nuclear hormone receptor and transcription factor found in a variety of tissues, including the gut, adipose tissue or the liver, as well as in most immunomodulatory processes of metabolism. (1-7)

1.25 (OH) 2D3 is produced in the skin after exposure to UV light or absorbed from a diet containing vitamin D-rich foods. (7) Low vitamin D levels or inactivating polymorphisms in VDR have been associated with inflammatory and metabolic disorders. (7)

Traditionally, vitamin D is known to regulate bone development and calcium homeostasis through its effects in the intestine, kidney, and bone. (7)

Vitamin D regulates calcium uptake in the gut and absorption in the kidney by activating transcellular calcium transport. (7)

Vitamin D is an essential nutrient that is not only important for bone health, but also beneficial for many other metabolic processes. (1-8)

The American Academy of Dermatology has declared UV radiation from the sun as a known carcinogen (8), which is why it may not be safe or effective to obtain vitamin D by exposure to sunlight. (2)

Therefore, physicians should inform patients at higher risk for vitamin D deficiency about how to adequately administer vitamin D through diet or supplementation (i.e older individuals, etc.). (2) Studies are currently underway to evaluate the effects of vitamin D supplementation and to determine the optimal serum level of vitamin D. (2, 9) Studies have also shown that recommendations for vitamin D supplementation should be individualized, or the recommended daily allowance for vitamin D for infants up to 12 months is 400 IU daily and 600 IU for children 1-18 years old , (2, 9)

This book summarizes important mechanisms of action of vitamin D in the human body based on current scientific findings.

Vitamin D metabolism:

Vitamin D3 (cholecalciferol) is absorbed through the diet (from fortified dairy products and fish oils) or synthesized in the skin by UV irradiation from 7-dehydrocholesterol. (24)

Vitamin D produced by 7-dehydrocholesterol depends on the intensity of UV irradiation, which varies with the season and latitude. (10)

Sunscreen and clothing have been reported to prevent the conversion of 7-dehydrocholesterol to vitamin D3. (11, 12)

In order to be biologically active and to influence mineral metabolism, as well as having effects on numerous other physiological functions, including the potential inhibition of the growth of cancer cells and protection against certain immune-mediated disorders, vitamin D is converted to its active form. (13, 14)

Vitamin D is transported in the blood through the vitamin D binding protein (DBP, a specific binding protein for vitamin D and its metabolites in the serum) to the liver. In the liver, vitamin D is hydroxylated by one or more cytochrome P450 vitamin D-25 hydroxylases (including CYP2R1, CYP2D11 and CYP2D25) resulting in the formation of 25-hydroxyvitamin D3 (25 (OH) D3). (24)

It has been suggested that CYP2R1 is the key enzyme for vitamin D hydroxylation since a homozygous mutation of the CYP2R1 gene was found in a patient with low levels of 25 (OH) D3 and classic symptoms of vitamin D deficiency. (15)

25 (OH) D3, the main circulatory form of vitamin D, is transported by the DBP to the kidney. (24) In the kidney, a member of the LDL receptor superfamily plays an essential role in the endocytic internalization of 25 (OH) D3. (16) In the proximal renal tubule, 25 (OH) D3 is hydroxylated to produce the vitamin D hormonally active 1,25-dihydroxyvitamin D3 (1,25 (OH) 2D3) responsible for most, if not all, of the biological effects of vitamin D. (24)

The cytochrome P450 monooxygenase 25 (OH) D 1α-hydroxylase (CYP27B1; 1α (OH) ase), which metabolizes 25 (OH) D3 to 1,25 (OH) 2 D3, is predominantly present in the kidney. (24) This enzyme is also found at extrarenal sites, including the placenta, monocytes and macrophages. (17-20, 24) As with all mitochondrial P450-containing enzymes, electrons are transferred via ferrodoxin from NADPH to NADPH-ferrodoxin reductase during the 1α (OH) -ase reaction. (24) Inactivating mutations in the 1α (OH) ase gene lead to vitamin D-dependent rickets despite normal intake of vitamin D, indicating the importance of the 1α (OH) ase enzyme. (21) Type 1 vitamin D-dependent rickets are characterized by growth disorders, hypocalcaemia, increased PTH, muscle weakness and radiological findings typical of rickets. (21, 22, 23)

Vitamin D is therefore a fat-soluble vitamin that can be obtained from food, as well as a prohormone that is formed by UV-B (UVB, 290-320 nm) from sunlight in the skin. (24-26) Vitamin D, as a precursor of a potent steroid hormone, is metabolized involving liver and kidney in two steps to synthesize a biologically active form, calcitriol, that binds to the vitamin D receptor (VDR). (25, 26)

The classical role of vitamin D is the regulation of calcium and phosphate metabolism, which is essential for bone remodeling. (27-31)

Extensive research in recent decades has shown, however, that low sun exposure and vitamin D deficiency are or could be associated with the increased risk of many other non-skeletal disorders. (27-31)

Vitamin D and bone metabolism:

The modern lifestyle limits our exposure to sunlight, which generates vitamin D in the skin. (32) Vitamin D is generated in all organisms from phytoplankton to mammals. (32)

Vitamin D is essential for mineral homeostasis and has a variety of non-skeletal functions, the most important of which for natural selection is a regulatory function in the innate immune system. (32)

The main effect of the active vitamin D metabolite 1,25 (OH) 2D is to stimulate the uptake of calcium from the intestine. (32) The consequences of vitamin D deficiency are secondary hyperparathyroidism and bone loss, which can lead to osteoporosis and bone fractures, mineralization defects that can lead to osteomalacia in the long run, and muscle weakness that can cause falls and broken bones. (33) Vitamin D status is related to bone mineral density and bone turnover. (33) Vitamin D supplementation can decrease bone turnover and increase bone mineral density. (33) Several randomized placebo-controlled studies with vitamin D and calcium showed a significant decrease in fracture incidence. (34, 33)

Subclinical vitamin D deficiency is more common and may be associated with osteoporosis and a higher incidence of falls or fractures. (2) The deposition of bone mineral begins in pregnancy, especially in the third trimester. (34, 35) Bone mass increases approximately 40-fold from birth to adulthood, reaching 90% of maximum bone mass at the end of the second decade of life. (36)

Childhood and adolescence are critical periods for the deposition of bone minerals. (37) A 2010 public health assessment showed that the intake of calcium in healthy children did not significantly reduce the frequency of fractures. (38) It was shown that a healthy, balanced diet that met the recommended calcium intake was superior to routine calcium intake. (39, 40) Due to the limited natural dietary sources of vitamin D and inadequate sun exposure in most children and adolescents, vitamin D supplementation is required. (2, 39)

Routine screening of 25 (OH) D levels, however, is not recommended, except for those at higher risk (eg, the elderly, obesity, chronic liver or kidney disease, etc.) or in children with poor growth, etc. (2), as well as eg in persons with elevated serum alkaline phosphatase, or those who spend very little time outdoors. (34, 39, 40)

Vitamin D and the immune system:

As mentioned above, VDRs are present throughout the body, including antigen-presenting cells, with known direct effects on innate and adaptive immunity. (2) The relationships between vitamin D and these diseases are discussed below: (2)

Tuberculosis (TB) – A link between vitamin D deficiency and TB has been reported. (41) It was reported in 2008 that UVB radiation had beneficial effects on TB therapy. (41) However, Martineau et al. concluded that taking vitamin D did not significantly improve clinical outcomes. (42)

Respiratory tract infections - In a prospective study by Camargo, an inverse relationship between 25 (OH) D levels in umbilical cord blood and the risk of upper respiratory infection was described. (43) A recent meta-analysis from 2017 showed a reduced incidence of acute respiratory infections after vitamin D supplementation. (45)

It has been reported that vitamin D, in addition to its classic effects on calcium and bone homeostasis, also performs other tasks. (46) The vitamin D receptor is expressed on immune cells (B cells, T cells and antigen presenting cells). (46) Vitamin D can modulate innate and adaptive immune responses, as reported previously. (46) It has been reported that vitamin D deficiency may be associated with increased autoimmunity and increased susceptibility to infection. (46)

There is increasing epidemiological evidence for a possible link between vitamin D deficiency and autoimmune diseases, including multiple sclerosis (MS), rheumatoid arthritis (RA), diabetes mellitus (DM), inflammatory bowel disease, and systemic lupus erythematosus (SLE) (47-50).

Vitamin D deficiency has also been implicated in various respiratory diseases, including otitis media. (64)

Vitamin D and cardiovascular disease and diabetes:

Study results suggest that patients with type 2 diabetes with vitamin D deficiency may be at higher risk for the development of cardiovascular disease and nephropathy. (65)

Vitamin D and MS:

The exact cause of multiple sclerosis (MS) is not yet known. (51) However, several factors have been identified that increase the risk of demyelinating central nervous system (CNS) disease and increase the severity of the disease. (51)

In addition to genetic determinants, environmental factors are now established that affect MS, which is of great interest, as some of these factors are relatively easy to change. (51) In this regard, it has been reported that low vitamin D status could be associated with increased relapse frequency and worsened disease in MS patients. (51)

Whether the supplementation of vitamin D in MS has a direct therapeutic benefit is still controversial. (51)

There is also evidence that excessive vitamin D treatment via the T-cell stimulating effect of secondary hypercalcaemia could have a negative impact on CNS demyelinating disease. (51)

Study results indicate that low vitamin D levels may be associated with an increased risk of cancer. (52) There are indications (53) that supplementation with vitamin D is associated with an increase in overall survival and a lower risk of relapse of myeloid, but not lymphoid, malignancies in transplant recipients. (52)

A possible association between vitamin D and immune regulation of the tumor microenvironment has also been reported by Liu et al. (52). Study results suggest that vitamin D has a regulatory effect on the NFκB signaling pathway. (55) In tumor stroma secretion of cytokines and prostaglandins is essential for the proliferation of cancer cells; vitamin D seems to have regulatory effects and to attenuate its secretion. (55)

On the other hand, Pawlik and co-workers (54) observed that vitamin D and its analogues modulate the prevalence of a given fraction of lymphocytes in the mouse mammary gland model. (54) This observation was accompanied by the modulation of the level of pro-tumorogenic cytokine in the serum. (54) It appears that the modulatory effects of vitamin D in the treatment of cancer may also include adverse effects that should be considered. (55)

A 2014 meta-study also showed that vitamin D deficiency is unlikely to affect carcinogenesis. (67, 52) Therefore, the authors did not recommend taking vitamin D supplements as a general precaution. (67, 52) Nevertheless, low levels of vitamin D may not be beneficial for the outcome of pre-existing cancer. (67, 52)

Vitamin D and the microbiome:

The microbiome is considered a newly discovered human organ. (56) It is crucial for the synthesis of vitamins and for obtaining otherwise inaccessible nutrients, the metabolism of xenobiotics, the storage of body fat, the renewal of intestinal epithelial cells and the maturation of the immune system. (56)

Vitamin D and its receptor (Vitamin D Receptor (VDR)) are known to regulate the microbiome in terms of health and disease. (7) There is evidence that vitamin D can regulate the inflammation of the gastrointestinal tract. (56) Further research in this area and the use of vitamin D as adjunctive therapy for patients with irritable bowel syndrome - IBD patients is required in this context. (56)

Vitamin D in context with ophthalmology:

There are epidemiological studies demonstrating that vitamin D levels and genetic variations influence the development of a variety of pathologies such as myopia, age-related macular degeneration, diabetic retinopathy, and others. (57)

Studies suggest that vitamin D plays a protective role in the eye, not least because of its described inflammatory modulating properties, which may be relevant in diseases such as age-related macular degeneration. (57-62) It remains to be seen what therapeutic benefits of vitamin D could be observed in the eye. (57)

Vitamin D in context with cardiovascular disease:

Although study findings also suggest that there is no beneficial effect of vitamin D supplementation on the incidence of cardiovascular disease or cancer, beneficial effects of vitamin D supplementation have also been observed: for persistence in taking statins in participants during a long-term therapy; and also in terms of bone mineral density and arterial function in subjects with low levels of 25-hydroxyvitamin D, as well as in lung function in smokers (especially in vitamin D deficiency). (66)

Vitamin D-unwanted effects:

Prolonged and inappropriate consumption of vitamin D supplements can lead to vitamin D poisoning. (63) One of the reasons why vitamin D supplements are considered safe is that they rarely increase serum vitamin D levels, even after repeated intravenous intake of extremely high doses of synthetic vitamin D analogues in toxic areas. (63)

Prolonged intake of vitamin D may, however, lead to hypercalcaemia, hypercalcuria and hyperphosphatemia, which are the first signs of vitamin D intoxication. (63) It is likely that dysregulation of calcium and phosphorus caused by exogenous vitamin D supplementation can lead to tissue and organ damage. (63)

Conclusion:

It is currently being discussed whether vitamin D should only be used as a dietary supplement, possibly for the prophylaxis or even for the treatment of multiple diseases. (55)

In view of the pleiotropic, modulatory effect of vitamin D, the serum level of 25-OH D3 should always be considered as an important diagnostic factor, especially in the case of vitamin D deficiency. (55)

Several clinical studies also showed beneficial effects of vitamin D supplementation on general human health and suggested that it could be used in the treatment of various diseases. (2, 55)

However, further extensive studies are needed to validate the potential benefits and safety of vitamin D in the clinic. (55)

For more detailed information on the topic of vitamin D reference is made to relevant literature (see references).

References:

1. Ran Zhang and Declan P Naughton.Vitamin D in health and disease: Current perspectives. Nutr J. 2010; 9: 65.
2. Chang SW, Lee HC. Vitamin D and health - The missing vitamin in humans. Pediatr Neonatol. 2019 Apr 17. pii: S1875-9572(18)30651-X.
3. O'Riordan, J.L. and Bijvoet, O.L. Rickets before the discovery of vitamin D. Bonekey Rep. 2014; 3: 478.
4. Mozolowski W. :Jedrzej Sniadecki (1768-1838) on the cure of rickets.. Nature. 1939; 143: 121–124.
5. Chick, H., Dalyell, E.J., Hume, M., Mackay, H.M.M., Henderson-Smith, H., and Wimberger, H. The aetiology of rickets in infants: prophylactic and curative observations at the Vienna University Kinderklinik. Lancet. 1922; 2: 7–11.
6. McCollum, E.V., Simmonds, N., Becker, J.E., and Shipley, P.G. Studies on the experimental demonstration of the existence of a vitamin which promotes calcium deposition. J Biol Chem. 1922;53: 293–312.
7. Jun Sun. Dietary Vitamin D, Vitamin D Receptor, and Microbiome. Curr Opin Clin Nutr Metab Care. 2018 Nov; 21(6): 471–474.
8. Vitamin D and UV exposure. American Academy of Dermatology. (Available at:) (Accessed December 1, 2018).
9. Dawodu, A. and Wagner, C.L. Mother-child vitamin D deficiency: an international perspective. Arch Dis Child. 2007; 92: 737–740.
10. Influence of season and latitude on the cutaneous synthesis of vitamin D3: exposure to winter sunlight in Boston and Edmonton will not promote vitamin D3 synthesis in human skin. Webb AR, Kline L, Holick MF. J Clin Endocrinol Metab. 1988 Aug; 67(2):373-8.
11. Sunscreens suppress cutaneous vitamin D3 synthesis. Matsuoka LY, Ide L, Wortsman J, MacLaughlin JA, Holick MF. J Clin Endocrinol Metab. 1987 Jun; 64(6):1165-8.
12. Clothing prevents ultraviolet-B radiation-dependent photosynthesis of vitamin D3. Matsuoka LY, Wortsman J,

Dannenberg MJ, Hollis BW, Lu Z, Holick MF. J Clin
Endocrinol Metab. 1992 Oct; 75(4):1099-103.
13. Enzymes involved in the activation and inactivation of
vitamin D. Prosser DE, Jones G. Trends Biochem Sci. 2004
Dec; 29(12):664-73.
14. Hydroxylase enzymes of the vitamin D pathway: expression,
function, and regulation. Omdahl JL, Morris HA, May BK.
Annu Rev Nutr. 2002; 22():139-66.
15. Genetic evidence that the human CYP2R1 enzyme is a key
vitamin D 25-hydroxylase. Cheng JB, Levine MA, Bell NH,
Mangelsdorf DJ, Russell DW. Proc Natl Acad Sci U S A.
2004 May 18; 101(20):7711-5.
16. An endocytic pathway essential for renal uptake and
activation of the steroid 25-(OH) vitamin D3. Nykjaer A,
Dragun D, Walther D, Vorum H, Jacobsen C, Herz J, Melsen
F, Christensen EI, Willnow TE. Cell. 1999 Feb 19;
96(4):507-15.
17. Weisman Y, Harell A, Edelstein S, et al. 1 alpha, 25-
Dihydroxyvitamin D3 and 24,25-dihydroxyvitamin D3 in
vitro synthesis by human decidua and
placenta. Nature. 1979;281:317–9.
18. Gray TK, Lester GE, Lorenc RS. Evidence for extra-renal 1
alpha-hydroxylation of 25-hydroxyvitamin D3 in
pregnancy. Science. 1979;204:1311–3.
19. Stoffels K, Overbergh L, Bouillon R, et al. Immune
regulation of 1alpha-hydroxylase in murine peritoneal
macrophages: unravelling the IFNgamma pathway. J Steroid
Biochem Mol Biol. 2007;103:567–71.
20. Esteban L, Vidal M, Dusso A. 1alpha-Hydroxylase
transactivation by gamma-interferon in murine macrophages
requires enhanced C/EBPbeta expression and activation. J
Steroid Biochem Mol Biol. 2004;89–90:131–7.
21. Kitanaka S, Takeyama K, Murayama A, et al. Inactivating
mutations in the 25-hydroxyvitamin D3 1alpha-hydroxylase
gene in patients with pseudovitamin D-deficiency rickets. N
Engl J Med. 1998;338:653–61.
22. Panda DK, Miao D, Tremblay ML, et al. Targeted ablation of
the 25-hydroxyvitamin D 1alpha -hydroxylase enzyme:

evidence for skeletal, reproductive, and immune dysfunction. Proc Natl Acad Sci U S A. 2001;98:7498–503.

23. 14. Dardenne O, Prud'homme J, Arabian A, et al. Targeted inactivation of the 25-hydroxyvitamin D(3)-1(alpha)-hydroxylase gene (CYP27B1) creates an animal model of pseudovitamin D-deficiency rickets. Endocrinology. 2001;142:3135–41.

24. Sylvia Christakos, Ph.D., Dare V. Ajibade, B.A., .Puneet Dhawan Ph.D., Adam J. Fechner, M.D.,[d] andLeila J. Mady, B.A. Vitamin D: Metabolism. Endocrinol Metab Clin North Am. 2010 Jun; 39(2): 243–253.

25. 1. Zhang R, Naughton DP. Vitamin D in health and disease: current perspectives. Nutr. J. 2010;9:65.

26. 2. Bouillon R, et al. Vitamin D and human health: lessons from vitamin D receptor null mice. Endocr. Rev. 2008;29:726–776.

27. 3. Bikle DD. Extraskeletal actions of vitamin D. Ann. N. Y Acad. Sci. 2016;1376:29–52.

28. 4. Holick MF. Sunlight and vitamin D for bone health and prevention of autoimmune diseases, cancers, and cardiovascular disease. Am. J. Clin. Nutr. 2004;80:1678S–1688S.

29. 5. Wang H, et al. Vitamin D and chronic diseases. Aging Dis. 2017;8:346–353.

30. E, Feldman BJ. The role of vitamin D in reducing cancer risk and progression. Nat. Rev. Cancer. 2014;14:342–357.

31. Sang-Min Jeonand Eun-Ae Shin· Exploring vitamin D metabolism and function in cancer. .Exp Mol Med 2018 Apr; 50(4): 20.

32. Hochberg Z, Hochberg I. Evolutionary Perspective in Rickets and Vitamin D. Front Endocrinol (Lausanne). 2019 May 15;10:306.

33. Lips P, van Schoor NM. Best Pract Res Clin Endocrinol Metab. 2011 Aug;25(4):585-91. doi: 10.1016/j.beem.2011.05.002. The effect of vitamin D on bone and osteoporosis.

34. Misra, M., Pacaud, D., Petryk, A., Collett-Solberg, P.F., and Kappy, M. Drug and therapeutics committee of the Lawson

Wilkins pediatric endocrine society. Vitamin D deficiency in children and its management: review of current knowledge and recommendations. Pediatrics. 2008; 122: 398–417.

35. Abrams, S.A. In utero physiology: role in nutrient delivery and fetal development for calcium, phosphorus, and vitamin D. Am J Clin Nutr. 2007; 85: 604S–607S.

36. Bachrach, L.K. Acquisition of optimal bone mass in childhood and adolescence. Trends Endocrinol Metab. 2001; 12: 22–28.

37. Golden, N.H., Abrams, S.A., and Committee on Nutrition. Optimizing bone health in children and adolescents. Pediatrics. 2014; 134: e1229–e1243.

38. Winzenberg, T.M., Powell, S., Shaw, K.A., and Jones, G. Vitamin D supplementation for improving bone mineral density in children. Cochrane Database Syst Rev. 2010; 10: CD006944.

39. Holick, M.F., Binkley, N.C., Bischoff-Ferrari, H.A., Gordon, C.M., Hanley, D.A., Heaney, R.P. et al.Evaluation, treatment, and prevention of vitamin D deficiency: an Endocrine Society clinical practice guideline. J Clin Endocrinol Metab. 2011; 96: 1911–1930.

40. Weydert, J.A. Vitamin D in children's health. Children. 2014; 1: 208–226.

41. Nnoaham, K.E. and Clarke, A. Low serum vitamin D levels and tuberculosis: a systemic review and meta-analysis. Int J Epidemiol. 2008; 37: 113–119.

42. Martineau, A.R., Timms, P.M., Bothamley, G.H., Hanifa, Y., Islam, K., Claxton, A.P. et al. High-dose vitamin D(3) during intensive-phase antimicrobial treatment of pulmonary tuberculosis: a double-blind randomised controlled trial. Lancet. 2011; 377: 242–250.

43. Camargo, C.A. Jr., Ingham, T., Wickens, K., Thadhani, R., Silvers, K.M., Epton, M.J. et al. Cord-blood 25-hydroxyvitamin D levels and risk of respiratory infection, wheezing, and asthma. Pediatrics. 2011;127: e180–e187.

44. Belderbos, M.E., Houben, M.L., Wilbrink, B., Lentjes, E., Bloemen, E.M., Kimpen, J.L. et al. Cord blood vitamin D deficiency is associated with respiratory syncytial virus bronchiolitis. Pediatrics. 2011; 127: e1513–e1520.

45. Martineau, A.R., Jolliffe, D.A., Hooper, R.L., Greenberg, L., Aloia, J.F., Bergman, P. et al. Vitamin D supplementation to prevent acute respiratory tract infection: systematic review and meta-analysis of individual participant data. BMJ. 2017; 356: i6583.

46. Cynthia Aranow, MD, Investigator. Vitamin D and the Immune System. J Investig Med. 2011 Aug; 59(6): 881–886.

47. Munger KL, et al. Serum 25-hydroxyvitamin D levels and risk of multiple sclerosis. JAMA. 2006;296(23):2832–8.

48. Littorin B, et al. Lower levels of plasma 25-hydroxyvitamin D among young adults at diagnosis of autoimmune type 1 diabetes compared with control subjects: results from the nationwide Diabetes Incidence Study in Sweden (DISS) Diabetologia. 2006;49(12):2847–52.

49. Merlino LA, et al. Vitamin D intake is inversely associated with rheumatoid arthritis: results from the Iowa Women's Health Study. Arthritis Rheum. 2004;50(1):72–7.

50. Fronczak CM, et al. In utero dietary exposures and risk of islet autoimmunity in children. Diabetes Care. 2003;26(12):3237–42.

51. Häusler D, Weber MS. Vitamin D Supplementation in Central Nervous System Demyelinating Disease-Enough Is Enough. Int J Mol Sci. 2019;20(1):218. Published 2019 Jan 8. doi:10.3390/ijms20010218.

52. The Anti-Inflammatory Effects of Vitamin D in Tumorigenesis. Liu W, Zhang L, Xu HJ, Li Y, Hu CM, Yang JY, Sun MY. Int J Mol Sci. 2018 Sep 13; 19(9).

53. Vitamin D: Effect on Haematopoiesis and Immune System and Clinical Applications. Medrano M, Carrillo-Cruz E, Montero I, Perez-Simon JA. Int J Mol Sci. 2018 Sep 8; 19(9).

54. Calcitriol and Its Analogs Establish the Immunosuppressive Microenvironment That Drives Metastasis in 4T1 Mouse Mammary Gland Cancer. Pawlik A, Anisiewicz A, Filip-Psurska B, Nowak M, Turlej E, Trynda J, Banach J, Gretkierewicz P, Wietrzyk J. Int J Mol Sci. 2018 Jul 20; 19(7).

55. Michal A. Zmijewski. Vitamin D and Human Health. Int J Mol Sci. 2019 Jan; 20(1): 145.

56. Tabatabaeizadeh SA, Tafazoli N, Ferns GA, Avan A, Ghayour-Mobarhan M. Vitamin D, the gut microbiome and inflammatory bowel disease. J Res Med Sci. 2018;23:75. Published 2018 Aug 23. doi:10.4103/jrms.JRMS_606_17.

57. Rose Y. Reins and . Alison M. McDermott. Vitamin D: Implications for Ocular Disease and Therapeutic Potential. Exp Eye Res. 2015 May; 134: 101–110.

58. Annamaneni S, Bindu CH, Reddy KP, Vishnupriya S. Association of vitamin D receptor gene start codon (Fok1) polymorphism with high myopia. Oman J. Ophthalmol. 2011;4:57–62.

59. Day S, Acquah K, Platt A, Lee PP, Mruthyunjaya P, Sloan FA. Association of vitamin D deficiency and age-related macular degeneration in medicare beneficiaries. Arch. Ophthalmol. 2012;130:1070–1071.

60. Bućan K, Ivanisević M, Zemunik T, Boraska V, Skrabić V, Vatavuk Z, Galetović D, Znaor L. Retinopathy and nephropathy in type 1 diabetic patients—association with polymorphysms of vitamin D-receptor, TNF, Neuro-D and IL-1 receptor 1 genes. Coll. Antropol. 2009;(33 Suppl 2):99–105.

61. Leyssens C, Verlinden L, Verstuyf A. Antineoplastic effects of 1,25(OH)2D3 and its analogs in breast, prostate and colorectal cancer. Endocr. Relat. Cancer. 2013;20:R31–R47.

62. Albert DM, Plum LA, Yang W, Marcet M, Lindstrom MJ, Clagett-Dame M, DeLuca HF. Responsiveness of human retinoblastoma and neuroblastoma models to a non-calcemic 19-nor Vitamin D analog. J. Steroid Biochem. Mol. Biol. 2005;97:165–172.

63. Razzaque MS. Can adverse effects of excessive vitamin D supplementation occur without developing hypervitaminosis D?. J Steroid Biochem Mol Biol. 2018 Jun;180:81-86.

64. Walker RE, Bartley J, Camargo CA Jr, Mitchell EA. Vitamin D and Otitis Media. Curr Allergy Asthma Rep. 2019 Jun 3;19(7):33.

65. Aljack HA, Abdalla MK, Idris OF, Ismail AM. Vitamin D deficiency increases risk of nephropathy and

cardiovascular diseases in Type 2 diabetes mellitus patients. J Res Med Sci. 2019 May 22;24:47.

66. Scragg, R.K.R. J Endocrinol Invest (2019).

67. B. Schöttker, R. Jorde u. a.: Vitamin D and mortality: meta-analysis of individual participant data from a large consortium of cohort studies from Europe and the United States. In: BMJ.Band 348, Juni 2014, S. g3656, doi:10.1136/bmj.g3656, PMID 24938302, PMC 4061380.

Impressum:

This book is translated from German: Vitamin D: Wirkungen auf den menschlichen Körper-Auf Basis aktueller wissenschaftlicher Erkenntnisse Kindle Ausgabe, Chrisotpher Schütze, Vienna, Asutria, 2019